The Essential Pressure Cooker Fish Recipes

Quick And Easy Delicious Dishes To Prepare At Home

Anissa E. Silvers

Sommario

Introduction

The Ninja Foodi multi-cooker is one of the home appliances that every person ought to have in their kitchen area. The device can replace four little tools: slow stove, air fryer, pressure cooker and dehydrator.

This cookbook consists of several of the recipes we have tried with the multi-cooker. The recipes vary from morning meal, side recipes, poultry, pork, soups, seafood, treats, and pasta. On top of that, we have actually compiled loads of vegetarian meals you should try. We developed these recipes considering beginners which's why the food preparation treatment is methodical. Besides, the meals are scrumptious, appreciate analysis.

Fish & Fries

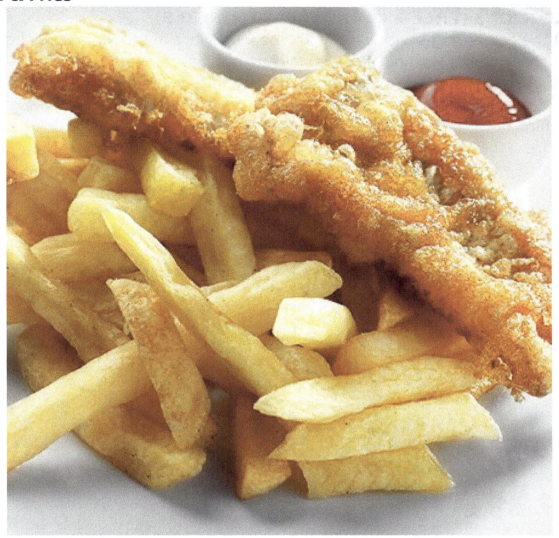

INGREDIENTS (4 Servings)

1 lb. potatoes, sliced into strips
 2 tablespoons olive oil
Salt and pepper to taste
1/4 cup all purpose flour
1 egg
2 tablespoons water
2/3 cup cornflakes, crushed
1 tablespoon Parmesan cheese, grated
1 lb. cod fillets

DIRECTIONS (PREP + COOK TIME: 30 MINUTES)

Coat the potato strips with oil, salt and pepper. Place in the Ninja Foodi basket. Seal the crisping lid and set it to air crisp. Cook at 400 degrees F for 10 minutes, stirring halfway through. While waiting, combine the flour with salt and pepper in one bowl. In another bowl, beat the egg and add water. In the third bowl, mix the cornflakes and Parmesan. Dip each fillet in the flour mixture. Then dip into the second and third bowls. Place in the Ninja Foodi basket. Seal the lid and choose air crisp function. Cook at 400 degrees for 10 minutes. Serving

Fish & Chips with Herb Sauce
INGREDIENTS (4 Servings)

2 potatoes, sliced into strips
Salt to taste
1/4 cup flour
1 egg
1 teaspoon Dijon mustard
3/4 cup seasoned panko bread crumbs
2 1/2 teaspoons olive oil
4 cod fish fillets
For the sauce:
1/4 cup light mayonnaise
2 tablespoons sour cream
2 tablespoons dill pickle, chopped
2 tablespoons red onion, chopped
1 tablespoon dill, chopped
1 tablespoon tarragon, chopped
2 teaspoons capers

DIRECTIONS (PREP + COOK TIME: 50 MINUTES)
Soak the potato strips in a bowl of water for 30 minutes. Drain the water and pat the potatoes dry using a paper towel. Place the potato strips in the Ninja Foodi basket. Seal the crisping lid and choose air crisp function. Cook at 360 degrees for 25 minutes, turning once or twice. Season with the salt. Put the flour in a bowl. Beat the egg and add the mustard in another bowl. Mix the oil and bread crumbs on a shallow plate. Coat the fish with the flour then the egg mixture, and then the oil with crumbs. Place in the basket. Cook at 360 degrees for 10 minutes. Mix all the ingredients for the sauce and serve with the fish and fries. Serving

. Fish Sticks
INGREDIENTS (4 Servings)

1 lb. cod, sliced into strips
1/2 cup tapioca starch
2 eggs
1 teaspoon dried dill
 Salt and pepper to taste
1 cup almond flour
1 teaspoon onion powder
1/2 teaspoon mustard powder
2 tablespoons avocado oil

DIRECTIONS (PREP + COOK TIME: 30 MINUTES)

Pat the cod fillet strips dry using paper towel. Place the tapioca starch in a bowl. In another bowl, beat the eggs. In a larger bowl, mix the dill, salt, pepper, almond flour, onion powder and mustard powder. Dip each strip in the first, second and third bowls. Coat the Ninja Foodi basket with the avocado oil. Place the fish strips inside. Cook at 390 degrees F for 5 minutes. Serving

Hot Prawns
INGREDIENTS (4 Servings)

1 teaspoon chili flakes
1 teaspoon chili powder
Salt and pepper to taste
12 king prawns
3 tablespoons mayonnaise
1 tablespoon ketchup
1 tablespoon wine vinegar

DIRECTIONS (PREP + COOK TIME: 15 MINUTES)
Combine all the spices in a bowl. Toss the prawns in the spice mixture. Place the prawns in the Ninja Foodi basket. Seal the crisping lid. Choose air crisp function. Cook at 360 degrees for 8 minutes. While waiting, mix the mayo, ketchup and vinegar. Serve with the prawns. Serving

Tuna Patties

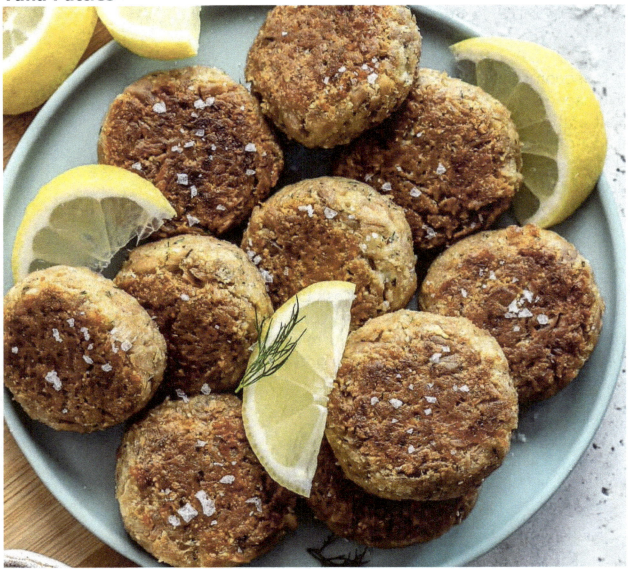

INGREDIENTS (2 Servings)

2 cans tuna flakes
1/2 tablespoon almond flour
1 teaspoon dried dill 1 tablespoon mayo
1/2 teaspoon onion powder
1 teaspoon garlic powder
Salt and pepper to taste
1 tablespoon lemon juice

DIRECTIONS (PREP + COOK TIME: 30 MINUTES)

Mix all the ingredients in a bowl. Form patties. Set the tuna patties on the Ninja Foodi basket. Seal the crisping lid. Set it to air crisp. Cook at 400 degrees for 10 minutes. Flip and cook for 5 more minutes. Serving

Crispy Cod Fish
INGREDIENTS (4 Servings)

4 cod fish fillets
Salt and sugar to taste
1 teaspoon sesame oil
250 ml water
5 tablespoons light soy sauce
1 teaspoon dark soy sauce
3 tablespoons oil
 5 slices ginger

DIRECTIONS (PREP + COOK TIME: 30 MINUTES)
Pat the cod fish fillets dry. Season with the salt, sugar and sesame oil. Marinate for 15 minutes. Set the Ninja Foodi to air crisp. Put the fish on top of the basket. Cook at 350 degrees F for 3 minutes. Flip and cook for 2 minutes. Take the fish out and set aside. Put the rest of the ingredients in the pot. Set it to sauté. Simmer and pour over the fish before serving. Serving

Heartfelt Sesame Fish
INGREDIENTS (4 Servings)

1 and ½ pound salmon fillet
1 teaspoon sesame seeds
1 teaspoon butter, melted
½ teaspoon salt
1 tablespoon apple cider vinegar
¼ teaspoon rosemary, dried

DIRECTIONS (PREP + COOK TIME: 16 MINUTES)
Take apple cider vinegar and spray it to the salmon fillets Then add dried rosemary, sesame seeds, butter and salt Mix them well. Take butter sauce and brush the salmon properly Place the salmon on the rack and lower the air fryer lid. Set the air fryer mode Cook the fish for 8 minutes at 360 F.Serve hot and enjoy!

Buttered Up Scallops
INGREDIENTS (4 Servings)

4 garlic cloves, minced
4 tablespoons rosemary, chopped
2 pounds sea scallops
12 cup butter
Salt and pepper to taste

DIRECTIONS (PREP + COOK TIME: 15 MINUTES)
Set your Ninja Foodi to Saute mode and add butter, rosemary, and garlic Saute for 1 minute. Add scallops, salt, and pepper Saute for 2 minutes. Lock Crisping lid and Crisp for 3 minutes at 350 degrees F. Serve and enjoy!

Lovely Air Fried Scallops
INGREDIENTS (4 Servings)

12 scallops
3 tablespoons olive oil
Salt and pepper to taste

DIRECTIONS (PREP + COOK TIME: 10 MINUTES)
Gently rub scallops with salt, pepper, and oil Transfer to your Ninja Foodie's insert, and place the insert in your Foodi Lock Air Crisping lid and cook for 4 minutes at 390 degrees F Half through, make sure to give them a nice flip and keep cooking. Serve warm and enjoy!

Garlic And Lemon Prawn Delight
INGREDIENTS (4 Servings)

2 tablespoons olive oil
1 pound prawns
2 tablespoons garlic, minced
2/3 cup fish stock
1 tablespoon butter
2 tablespoons lemon juice
1 tablespoon lemon zest
Salt and pepper to taste

DIRECTIONS (PREP + COOK TIME: 10 MINUTES)
Set your Ninja Foodi to Saute mode and add butter and oil, let it heat up Stir in remaining ingredients. Lock lid and cook on LOW pressure for 5 minutes Quick release pressure. Serve and enjoy!

Lovely Panko Cod

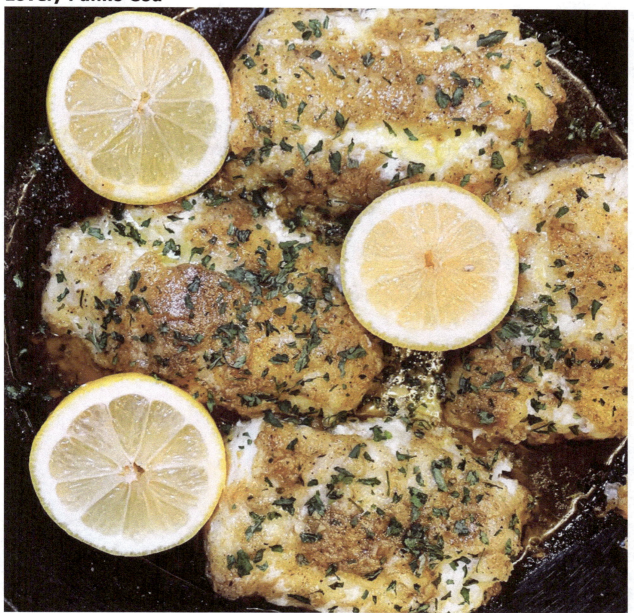

INGREDIENTS (6 Servings)

2 uncooked cod fillets,
6 ounces each
3 teaspoons kosher salt
¾ cup panko bread crumbs
2 tablespoons butter, melted
¼ cup fresh parsley, minced

1 lemon.
Zested and juiced

DIRECTIONS (PREP + COOK TIME: 20 MINUTES)

Pre-heat your Ninja Foodi at 390 degrees F and place Air Crisper basket inside Season cod and salt Take a bowl and add bread crumbs, parsley, lemon juice, zest, butter, and mix well Coat fillets with the bread crumbs mixture and place fillets in your Air Crisping basket Lock Air Crisping lid and cook on Air Crisp mode for 15 minutes at 360 degrees F Serve and enjoy!

Ranch Warm Fillets
INGREDIENTS (4 Servings)

¼ cup panko
½ packet ranch dressing mix powder
1 and ¼ tablespoons vegetable oil
1 egg beaten
2 tilapia fillets
A garnish of herbs and chilies

DIRECTIONS (PREP + COOK TIME: 18 MINUTES)
Pre-heat your Ninja Foodi with the Crisping Basket inside at 350 degrees
F Take a bowl and mix in ranch dressing and panko Beat eggs in a shallow
bowl and keep it on the side Dip fillets in the eggs, then in the panko
mix Place fillets in your Ninja Foodie's insert and transfer insert to Ninja
Foodi Lock Air Crisping Lid and Air Crisp for 13 minutes at 350 degrees
F Garnish with chilies and herbs. Enjoy!

Kale And Salmon Delight
INGREDIENTS (4 Servings)

1 lemon, juiced
2 salmon fillets
¼ cup extra virgin olive oil
1 teaspoon Dijon mustard
4 cups kale, thinly sliced, ribs removed
1 teaspoon salt
1 avocado, diced
1 cup pomegranate seeds
1 cup walnuts, toasted
1 cup goat parmesan cheese, shredded

DIRECTIONS (PREP + COOK TIME: 15 MINUTES)
Season salmon with salt and keep it on the side. Place a trivet in your Ninja Foodi Place salmon over the trivet. Lock lid and cook on HIGH pressure for 15 minutes Release pressure naturally over 10 minutes. Transfer salmon to a serving platter Take a bowl and add kale, season with salt Take another bowl and make the dressing by adding lemon juice, Dijon mustard, olive oil, and red wine vinegar. Season kale with dressing and add diced avocado, pomegranate seeds, walnuts and cheese. Toss and serve with the fish. Enjoy!

Lemon And Pepper Salmon Delight
INGREDIENTS (4 Servings)

¾ cup of water
Sprigs of parsley, basil, tarragon
1 pound salmon, skin on
3 teaspoons ghee
¾ teaspoon salt
½ teaspoon pepper
 ½ lemon, sliced
1 red bell pepper, julienned
1 carrot, julienned

DIRECTIONS (PREP + COOK TIME: 11 MINUTES)
Set your Ninja Foodi to Saute mode and add water and herbs Place a steamer rack and add the salmon. Drizzle ghee on top of the salmon Season with pepper and salt. Cover lemon slices on top Lock up the lid and cook on HIGH pressure for 3 minutes Release the pressure naturally over 10 minutes Transfer the salmon to a platter. Add veggies to your pot and set the pot to Saute mode Cook for 1-2 minutes. Serve the cooked vegetables with salmon. Enjoy!

Ranch Fish Fillet
INGREDIENTS (4 Servings)

3/4 cup bread crumbs
1 packet dry ranch dressing mix 2
1/2 tablespoons vegetable oil
2 eggs, beaten 4 fish fillets

DIRECTIONS (PREP + COOK TIME: 20 MINUTES)
Combine the bread crumbs and ranch mix in a bowl. Pour in the oil. Dip each fish fillet into the egg and cover with the crumb mixture. Place in the Ninja Foodi basket. Seal the lid. Select air crisp function.Cook at 360 degrees F for 12 minutes, flipping halfway through. Serving

Paprika Salmon
INGREDIENTS (2 Servings)

2 salmon fillets
2 teaspoons avocado oil
2 teaspoons paprika
Salt and pepper to taste

DIRECTIONS (PREP + COOK TIME: 15 MINUTES)
Coat the salmon with oil. Season with salt, pepper and paprika. Place in the Ninja Foodi basket. Set it to air crisp function. Seal the crisping lid. Cook at 390 degrees for 7 minutes. Serving

Southern Fried Fish Fillet

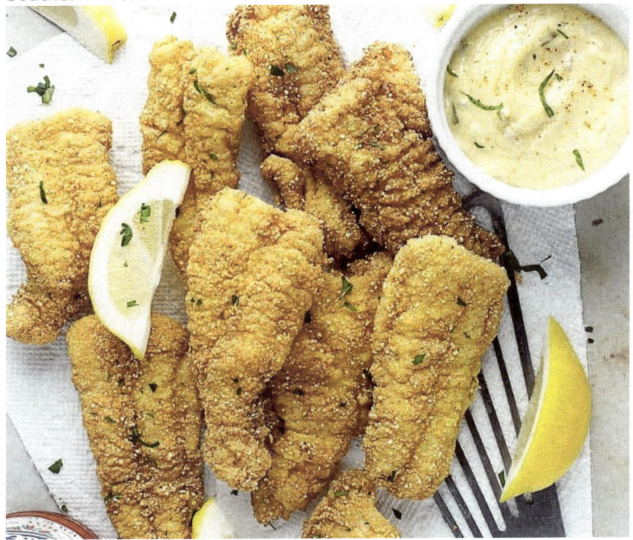

INGREDIENTS (4 Servings)

2 lb. white fish fillet
1 cup low fat milk
1 lemon slice
1/2 cup mustard
1/2 cup cornmeal
1/4 cup all purpose flour
2 tablespoons dried parsley flakes
Salt and pepper to taste
1/4 teaspoon chili powder

1/4 teaspoon garlic powder
1/4 teaspoon onion powder
1/4 teaspoon cayenne pepper

DIRECTIONS (PREP + COOK TIME: 30 MINUTES)

Place the fish fillet in a bowl. Pour the milk over the fish fillet. Squeeze lemon slice over the fish. Marinate for 15 minutes. Spread the mustard on the fish fillets. In another bowl, mix the rest of the ingredients. Coat the fish fillets with the cornmeal mixture. Place on the Ninja Foodi basket. Set it to air crisp. Seal the crisping lid. Cook at 390 degrees for 10 minutes.Flip the fillets and cook for 5 more minutes. Serving

Fish Fillet with Pesto Sauce
INGREDIENTS (3 Servings)

3 white fish fillets
1 tablespoon olive oil
Salt and pepper to taste
2 cups fresh basil leaves
 2 cloves garlic, crushed
2 tablespoons pine nuts
1 tablespoon Parmesan cheese, grated
1 cup olive oil

DIRECTIONS (PREP + COOK TIME: 20 MINUTES)

Coat the fish fillets with 1 tablespoon of olive oil. Season with the salt and pepper. Place in the Ninja Foodi basket. Cook at 320 degrees for 8 minutes. While waiting, mix the remaining ingredients in a food processor. Pulse until smooth. Spread the pesto sauce on both sides of the fish before serving. Serving

Coconut Shrimp
INGREDIENTS (4 Servings)

1/2 cup all purpose flour
1 1/2 teaspoons black pepper
2 eggs
1/3 cup panko bread crumbs
2/3 cup unsweetened coconut flakes
12 oz. shrimp, peeled and deveined
Cooking spray
Salt and pepper to taste
1/4 cup honey
1/4 cup lime juice

DIRECTIONS (PREP + COOK TIME: 20 MINUTES)
Mix the flour and black pepper in a bowl. In another bowl, beat the egg. In the third bowl, mix the bread crumbs and coconut flakes. Dip each of the shrimp in the first, second and third bowls. Place in the Ninja Foodi basket. Set it to air crisp.Cover the crisping lid. Cook at 400 degrees F for 8 minutes, turn halfway through. Season with the salt and pepper. Mix the remaining ingredients and serve with the shrimp. Serving

Crispy Shrimp
INGREDIENTS (4 Servings)

1 lb. shrimp, peeled and deveined
2 eggs
1/2 cup bread crumbs
1/2 cup onion, diced
1 teaspoon ginger
1 teaspoon garlic powder
Salt and pepper to taste

DIRECTIONS (PREP + COOK TIME: 20 MINUTES)

In one bowl, beat the two eggs. In another bowl, put the rest of the ingredients.Dip the shrimp first in the eggs and then in the spice mixture. Place in the Ninja Foodi basket.Seal the crisping lid. Choose air crisp function. Cook at 350 degrees for 10 minutes. Serving

Salt and Pepper Shrimp
INGREDIENTS (4 Servings)

2 teaspoons peppercorns
1 teaspoon salt
1 teaspoons sugar
1 lb. shrimp
3 tablespoons rice flour
2 tablespoons oil

DIRECTIONS (PREP + COOK TIME: 20 MINUTES)

Set the Ninja Foodi to sauté. Roast the peppercorns for 1 minute. Let them cool. Crush the peppercorns and add the salt and sugar. Coat the shrimp with this mixture and then with flour. Sprinkle oil on the Ninja Foodi basket. Place the shrimp on top. Cook at 350 degrees for 10 minutes, flipping halfway through. Serving

Lemon Garlic Shrimp
INGREDIENTS (4 Servings)

1 lb. shrimp, peeled and deveined
1 tablespoon olive oil
4 cloves garlic, minced
1 tablespoon lemon juice
Salt to taste

DIRECTIONS (PREP + COOK TIME: 40 MINUTES)
Mix the olive oil, salt, lemon juice and garlic.Toss shrimp in the mixture. Marinate for 15 minutes. Place the shrimp in the Ninja Foodi basket. Seal the crisping lid. Select the air crisp setting. Cook at 350 degrees for 8 minutes. Flip and cook for 2 more minutes. Serving

Crispy Fish Nuggets

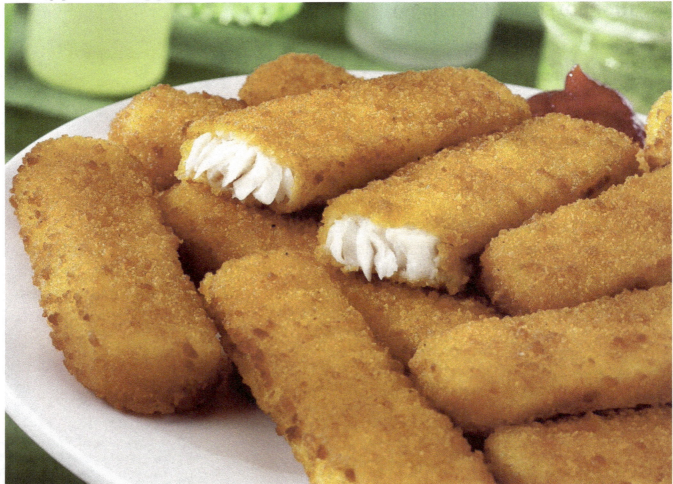

INGREDIENTS (4 Servings)

1 lb. cod fillet, sliced into
8 pieces Salt and pepper to taste
1/2 cup flour
1 tablespoon egg with
1 teaspoon water
1 cup bread crumbs
1 tablespoon vegetable oil

DIRECTIONS (PREP + COOK TIME: 30 MINUTES)
Season the fish with salt and pepper. Cover with the flour. Dip the fish in the
egg wash and into the bread crumbs. Place the fish nuggets in the Ninja Foodi

basket. Set it to air crisp function. Seal with the crisping lid. Cook at 360 degrees for 15 minutes. Serving

Awesome Sock-Eye Salmon
INGREDIENTS (4 Servings)

4 sockeye salmon fillets
1 teaspoon Dijon mustard
¼ teaspoon garlic, minced
¼ teaspoon onion powder
¼ teaspoon lemon pepper
½ teaspoon garlic powder
¼ teaspoon salt
2 tablespoons olive oil
1 and ½ cup of water

DIRECTIONS (PREP + COOK TIME: 10 MINUTES)
Take a bowl and add mustard, lemon juice, onion powder, lemon pepper, garlic powder, salt, olive oil. Brush spice mix over salmon Add water to Instant Pot. Place rack and place salmon fillets on rack Lock lid and cook on LOW pressure for 7 minutes Quick release pressure .Serve and enjoy!

Awesome Cherry Tomato Mackerel
INGREDIENTS (4 Servings)

4 Mackerel fillets
¼ teaspoon onion powder
¼ teaspoon lemon powder
 ¼ teaspoon garlic powder
½ teaspoon salt
2 cups cherry tomatoes
3 tablespoons melted butter
1 and ½ cups of water
1 tablespoon black olives

DIRECTIONS (PREP + COOK TIME: 12 MINUTES)
Grease baking dish and arrange cherry tomatoes at the bottom of the dish Top with fillets sprinkle all spices. Drizzle melted butter over Add water to your Ninja Foodi Lower rack in Ninja Foodi and place baking dish on top of the rack Lock lid and cook on LOW pressure for 7 minutes . Quick release pressure. Serve and enjoy!

Packets Of Lemon And Dill Cod
INGREDIENTS (4 Servings)

2 tilapia cod fillets Salt, pepper and garlic powder to taste
2 sprigs fresh dill
4 slices lemon
2 tablespoons butter

DIRECTIONS (PREP + COOK TIME: 20 MINUTES) Layout 2 large squares of parchment paper Place fillet in center of each parchment square and season with salt, pepper and garlic powder On each fillet, place 1 sprig of dill, 2 lemon slices, 1 tablespoon butter Place trivet at the bottom of your Ninja Foodi. Add 1 cup water into the pot Close parchment paper around fillets and fold to make a nice seal Place both packets in your pot . Lock lid and cook on HIGH pressure for 5 minutes Quick release pressure . Serve and enjoy!

Adventurous Sweet And Sour Fish
INGREDIENTS (4 Servings)

2 drops liquid stevia
¼ cup butter
1 pound fish chunks
1 tablespoon vinegar
Salt and pepper to taste

DIRECTIONS (PREP + COOK TIME: 16 MINUTES)
Set your Ninja Foodi to Saute mode and add butter, let it melt Add fish chunks and Saute for 3 minutes. Add stevia, salt, and pepper, stir Lock Crisping Lid and cook on "Air Crisp" mode for 3 minutes at 360 degrees F Serve once done and enjoy!

Lovely Carb Soup
INGREDIENTS (4 Servings)

1 cup crab meat, cubed
1 tablespoon garlic, minced
Salt as needed Red chili flakes as needed
3 cups vegetable broth
1 teaspoon salt

DIRECTIONS (PREP + COOK TIME: 6-7 hours and 5 MINUTES)
Coat the crab cubes in lime juice and let them sit for a while Add the all ingredients (including marinated crab meat) to your Ninja Foodi and lock lid Cook on SLOW COOK MODE (MEDIUM) for 3 hours Let it sit for a while Unlock lid and set to Saute mode, simmer the soup for 5 minutes more on LOW Stir and check to season. Enjoy!

The Rich Guy Lobster And Butter

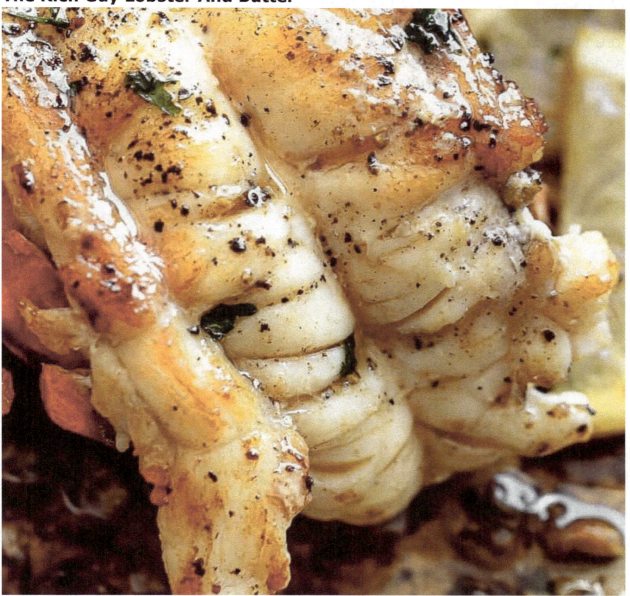

INGREDIENTS (4 Servings)

6 Lobster Tails
4 garlic cloves,
¼ cup butter

DIRECTIONS (PREP + COOK TIME: 20 MINUTES)

Preheat the Ninja Foodi to 400 degrees F at first Open the lobster tails gently by using kitchen scissors Remove the lobster meat gently from the shells but keep it inside the shells Take a plate and place it Add some butter in a pan and allow it melt Put some garlic cloves in it and heat it over medium-low heat Pour the garlic butter mixture all over the lobster tail meat Let the fryer to broil the lobster at 130 degrees F Remove the lobster meat from Ninja Foodi and set aside Use a fork to pull out the lobster meat from the shells entirely Pour some garlic butter over it if needed. Serve and enjoy!

Salmon Paprika
INGREDIENTS (4 Servings)

2 wild caught salmon fillets,
1 to 1 and ½ inches thick
2 teaspoons avocado oil
2 teaspoons paprika
Salt and pepper to taste
Green herbs to garnish

DIRECTIONS (PREP + COOK TIME: 12 MINUTES)
Season salmon fillets with salt, pepper, paprika, and olive oil Place Crisping basket in your Ninja Foodi, and pre-heat your Ninja Foodie at 390 degrees F Place insert insider your Foodi and place the fillet in the insert, lock Air Crisping lid and cook for 7 minutes. Once done, serve the fish with herbs on top. Enjoy!

Heartfelt Air Fried Scampi
INGREDIENTS (4 Servings)

4 tablespoons butter
1 tablespoon lemon juice
1 tablespoon garlic, minced
2 teaspoons red pepper flakes
 1 tablespoon chives, chopped
1 tablespoon basil leaves, minced
2 tablespoons chicken stock
1 pound defrosted shrimp

DIRECTIONS (PREP + COOK TIME: 10 MINUTES)
Set your Foodi to Saute mode and add butter, let the butter melt and add red pepper flakes and garlic, Saute for 2 minutes Transfer garlic to crisping basket, add remaining ingredients (including shrimp) to the basket Return basket back to the Ninja Foodi and lock the Air Crisping lid, cook for 5 minutes at 390 degrees F. Once done, serve with a garnish of fresh basil

Alaskan Cod Divine
INGREDIENTS (4 Servings)

1 large fillet, Alaskan Cod (Frozen)
1 cup cherry tomatoes
Salt and pepper to taste
Seasoning as you need
2 tablespoons butter
Olive oil as needed

DIRECTIONS (PREP + COOK TIME: 20 MINUTES)

Take an ovenproof dish small enough to fit inside your pot Add tomatoes to the dish, cut large fish fillet into 2-3 serving pieces and lay them on top of tomatoes. Season with salt, pepper, and your seasoning Top each fillet with 1 tablespoon butter and drizzle olive oil Add 1 cup of water to the pot.Place trivet to the Ninja Foodi and place dish on the trivet Lock lid and cook on HIGH pressure for 9 minutes.Release pressure naturally over 10 minutes Serve and enjoy!

Breathtaking Cod Fillets
INGREDIENTS (4 Servings)

1 pound frozen cod fish fillets
2 garlic cloves, halved
1 cup chicken broth
½ cup packed parsley
2 tablespoons oregano
2 tablespoons almonds, sliced
½ teaspoon paprika

DIRECTIONS (PREP + COOK TIME: 20 MINUTES)

Take the fish out of the freezer and let it defrost Take a food processor and stir in garlic, oregano, parsley, paprika, 1 tablespoon almond and process. Set your Ninja Foodi to "SAUTE" mode and add olive oil, let it heat up Add remaining almonds and toast, transfer to a towel. Pour broth in a pot and add herb mixture Cut fish into 4 pieces and place in a steamer basket, transfer steamer basket to the pot Lock lid and cook on HIGH pressure for 3 minutes. Quick release pressure once has done Serve steamed fish by pouring over the sauce.Enjoy!

Fresh Steamed Salmon
INGREDIENTS (4 Servings)

2 salmon fillets
¼ cup onion, chopped
2 stalks green onion stalks, chopped
1 whole egg
Almond meal
Salt and pepper to taste
2 tablespoons olive oil

DIRECTIONS (PREP + COOK TIME: 10 MINUTES)

 Add a cup of water to your Ninja Foodi and place a steamer rack on top Place the fish. Season the fish with salt and pepper and lock up the lid Cook on HIGH pressure for 3 minutes. Once done, quick release the pressure Remove the fish and allow it to cool Break the fillets into a bowl and add egg, yellow and green onions Add ½ a cup of almond meal and mix with your hand. Divide the mixture into patties Take a large skillet and place it over medium heat. Add oil and cook the patties.Enjoy!

Coconut Baked Trout

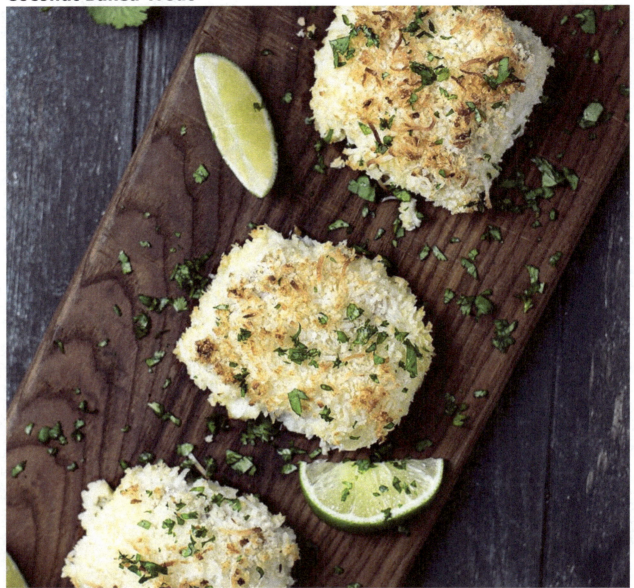

INGREDIENTS (4 Servings)

2 tablespoons parsley, chopped
2 teaspoons olive oil
2 teaspoons garlic, minced
4 trout fillets, skinless and boneless
1/2 cup coconut milk
Black pepper (ground) and salt to taste

DIRECTIONS (Prep + Cook Time: 20-25 minutes)

Take a baking pan, grease it with some cooking spray, vegetable oil, or butter. Add all the ingredients and combine well. Take Ninja Foodi multi-cooker, arrange it over a cooking platform, and open the top lid. In the pot, add water and place a reversible rack inside the pot. Place the pan over the rack. Seal the multi-cooker by locking it with the Crisping Lid, ensure to keep the pressure release valve locked/sealed. Select "BAKE/ROAST" mode and adjust the 380°F temperature level. Then after, set timer to 15 minutes and press "STOP/START," it will start the cooking process by building up inside pressure. When the timer goes off, quickly release pressure by adjusting the pressure valve to the VENT. After pressure gets released, open the Crisping Lid. Serve warm.

Wholesome Broccoli Shrimp
INGREDIENTS (4 Servings)

3 garlic cloves, minced
¼ cup white wine
2 tablespoons unsalted butter
1 shallot, minced
½ cup chicken stock
½ teaspoon Black pepper (ground)
1 ½ pounds frozen shrimp, thawed
Juice of ½ lemon
½ teaspoon of sea salt
1 large head broccoli, cut into florets

DIRECTIONS (Prep + Cook Time: 7-12 minutes)

Take Ninja Foodi multi-cooker, arrange it over a cooking platform, and open the top lid. In the pot, add the butter, Select "SEAR/SAUTÉ" mode and select "MD: HI" pressure level. Press "STOP/START." After about 4-5 minutes, the butter will melt. Add the shallots and cook (while stirring) until they become softened and translucent for 2-3 minutes. Add the garlic and cook for 1 minute. Add the wine and stir gently. Mix in the chicken stock, lemon juice, salt, pepper, broccoli, and shrimp. Seal the multi-cooker by locking it with the pressure lid, ensure to keep the pressure release valve locked/sealed. Select "PRESSURE" mode and select the "HI" pressure level. Then after, set timer to 1 minute and press "STOP/START," it will start the cooking process by building up inside pressure. When the timer goes off, quickly release pressure by adjusting the pressure valve to the VENT. After pressure gets released, open the pressure lid. Serve warm.

Cod Sandwich
INGREDIENTS (4 Servings)

1 cup cornstarch
1 cup all-purpose flour
2 eggs
8 ounces ale
1 teaspoon sea salt
1 teaspoon black pepper (ground)
½ tablespoon chili powder
1 tablespoon ground cumin
Tartar sauce
8 slices sandwich bread
4 (5-6 ounce) cod fillets, cut into 16 half-inch strips

DIRECTIONS (Prep + Cook Time: 20-25 minutes)
In a mixing bowl, whisk the eggs and beer. In another bowl, whisk the cornstarch, flour, chili powder, cumin, salt, and pepper. First, coat the cod fillets with the egg mixture and then with the flour mixture. Take Ninja Foodi multi-cooker, arrange it over a cooking platform, and open the top lid. In the pot, place the Crisping Basket, coat it with some cooking oil. In the basket, add the fillets. Seal the multi-cooker by locking it with the crisping lid, ensure to keep the pressure release valve locked/sealed. Select the "AIR CRISP" mode and adjust the 375°F temperature level. Then after, set timer to 15 minutes and press "STOP/START," it will start the cooking process by building up inside pressure. When the timer goes off, quickly release pressure by adjusting the pressure valve to the VENT. After pressure gets released, open the Crisping Lid. Arrange four bread slices and spread the tartar sauce over, place the fillets, and add remaining slices on top. Serve fresh.

Crispy Crabby Patties
INGREDIENTS (4 Servings)

1 shallot, minced
¼ cup mayonnaise, low carb
12 ounces lump crabmeat
¼ cup parsley, minced
2 tablespoons Dijon mustard
2 tablespoons almond flour
1 lemon, zest
1 egg, beaten
Pepper and salt as needed

DIRECTIONS (Prep + Cook Time: 15-20 minutes)
Take a mixing bowl and add all ingredients, mix well and prepare 4 meat from the mixture Pre-heat Ninja Foodi by pressing the "AIR CRISP" option and setting it to "375 Degrees F" and timer to 10 minutes Let it pre-heat until you hear a beep Transfer patties to cooking basket and let them cook for 5 minutes, flip and cook for 5 minutes more Serve and enjoy once done!

Baked Parmesan Fish
INGREDIENTS (3 Servings)

¼ teaspoon salt
¾ cup breadcrumbs
¼ cup parmesan cheese, grated
¼ teaspoon ground dried thyme
¼ cup butter, melted
1-pound haddock fillets
¾ cup milk

DIRECTIONS (Prep + Cook Time: 18-23 minutes)
Coat fish fillets in milk, season with salt and keep it on the side Take a mixing bowl and add breadcrumbs, parmesan, cheese, thyme and combine well Coat fillets in bread crumb mixture Pre-heat Ninja Foodi by pressing the "BAKE" option and setting it to "325 Degrees F" and timer to 13 minutes Let it pre-heat until you hear a beep Arrange fish fillets directly over Grill Grate, lock lid and cook for 8 minutes, flip and cook for the remaining time Serve and enjoy!

Crispy Garlic Mackerel
INGREDIENTS (4 Servings)

1 teaspoon garlic powder
1 teaspoon cumin, ground
4 mackerel fillets, boneless
1 tablespoon canola oil
Juice of 1 lime
Black pepper (ground) and salt to taste

DIRECTIONS (Prep + Cook Time: 17-22 minutes)
Take Ninja Foodi multi-cooker, arrange it over a cooking platform, and open the top lid.   In the pot, arrange a reversible rack and place the Crisping Basket over the rack. In the basket, add the fish and other ingredients, combine well.   Seal the multi-cooker by locking it with the crisping lid, ensure to keep the pressure release valve locked/sealed. Select the "AIR CRISP" mode and adjust the 370°F temperature level. Then after, set timer to 12 minutes and press "STOP/START," it will start the cooking process by building up inside pressure. Flip the fish after 6 minutes.   When the timer goes off, quickly release pressure by adjusting the pressure valve to the VENT. After pressure gets released, open the Crisping Lid. Serve warm with chopped salad greens (optional).

Salmon Rice Meal

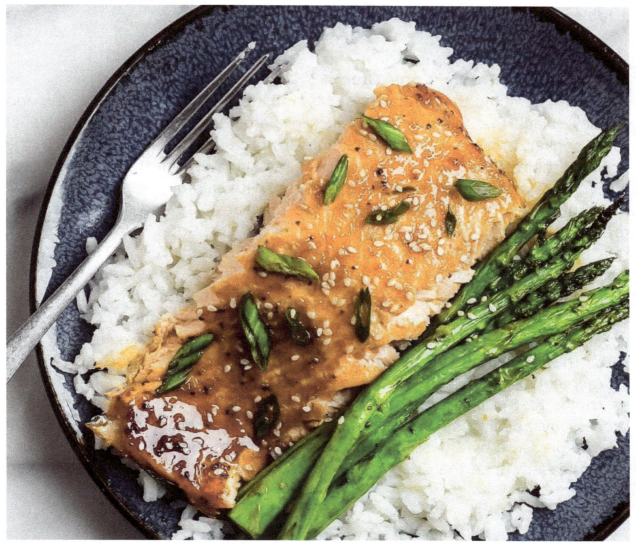

INGREDIENTS (4 Servings)

⅓ cup dry cranberries
⅓ cup slivered almonds
1 ½ cups long-grain white rice, rinsed
1 ½ cups water
Kosher salt
4 (4-ounce) salmon fillets
⅓ cup panko bread crumbs
1 tablespoon honey
⅓ cup dry roasted sunflower seeds

¼ cup Dijon mustard
1 tablespoon minced parsley

DIRECTIONS (Prep + Cook Time: 15-20 minutes)

In a bowl, combine the sunflower seeds, mustard, bread crumbs, honey, and parsley. Place the salmon fillets over an aluminum foil. Take Ninja Foodi multi-cooker, arrange it over a cooking platform, and open the top lid. In the pot, add the rice, salt, water, cranberries, and almonds; stir the mixture. Place a reversible rack inside the pot. Place the foil with salmon fillets over it. Seal the multi-cooker by locking it with the pressure lid; ensure to keep the pressure release valve locked/sealed. Select "PRESSURE" mode and select the "HI" pressure level. Then, set timer to 2 minutes and press "STOP/START"; it will start the cooking process by building up inside pressure. When the timer goes off, naturally release inside pressure for about 8-10 minutes. Then, quick-release pressure by adjusting the pressure valve to the VENT. Add the sesame mixture over the salmon fillets. Seal the multi-cooker by locking it with the Crisping Lid; ensure to keep the pressure release valve locked/sealed. Select "BROIL" mode and select the "HI" pressure level. Then, set timer to 8 minutes and press "STOP/START"; it will start the cooking process by building up inside pressure. When the timer goes off, quickly release pressure by adjusting the pressure valve to the VENT. After pressure gets released, open the Crisping Lid. Fluff the rice and serve with the cooked salmon.

Shrimp Cod Stew
INGREDIENTS (5-6 Servings)

1 fennel bulb, tops removed and bulb diced
3 garlic cloves, minced
2 tablespoons extra-virgin olive oil
1 yellow onion, diced
1 cup dry white wine
1 pound medium (21-30 count) shrimp, peeled and deveined
1 pound raw white fish (cod or haddock), cubed
2 (14.5-ounce) cans fire-roasted tomatoes
2 cups chicken stock
Salt
Black pepper (finely ground)
Fresh basil

DIRECTIONS (Prep + Cook Time: 45-50 minutes) Take Ninja Foodi multi-cooker, arrange it over a cooking platform and open the top lid. In the pot, add the oil; Select "SEAR/SAUTÉ" mode and select "MD:HI" pressure level. Press "STOP/START". After about 4-5 minutes, the oil will start simmering. Add the onions, fennel, garlic, and cook (while stirring) until become softened and translucent for 2-3 minutes. Add the white wine, roasted tomatoes and chicken stock. Simmer the mixture for 25-30 minutes. Add the shrimp and white fish. Stir-cook for 10 more minutes until the fish is cooked well. Season with salt and pepper. Serve with the basil leaves on top.

Hearty Swordfish Meal
INGREDIENTS (4 Servings)

5 swordfish fillets
½ a cup of melted clarified butter
6 garlic cloves, chopped
1 tablespoon black pepper

DIRECTIONS (PREP + COOK TIME: 150 MINUTES) Take a mixing bowl and add garlic, clarified butter, black pepper Take a parchment paper and add the fillet. Cover and wrap the fish Keep repeating until the fillets are wrapped up Transfer wrapped fish to Ninja Foodi pot and lock lid Allow them to cook for 2 and a ½ hour at high pressure. Release the pressure naturally Serve and enjoy!

Awesome Sock-Eye Salmon
INGREDIENTS (4 Servings)

4 sockeye salmon fillets
1 teaspoon Dijon mustard
¼ teaspoon garlic, minced
¼ teaspoon onion powder
 ¼ teaspoon lemon pepper
½ teaspoon garlic powder
¼ teaspoon salt
2 tablespoons olive oil
1 and ½ cup of water

DIRECTIONS (PREP + COOK TIME: 10 MINUTES) Take a bowl and add mustard, lemon juice, onion powder, lemon pepper, garlic powder, salt, olive oil. Brush spice mix over salmon Add water to Instant Pot. Place rack and place salmon fillets on rack Lock lid and cook on LOW pressure for 7 minutes Quick release pressure .Serve and enjoy!

Lovely Air Fried Scallops
INGREDIENTS (4 Servings)

12 scallops
3 tablespoons olive oil
Salt and pepper to taste

DIRECTIONS (PREP + COOK TIME: 10 MINUTES)
Gently rub scallops with salt, pepper, and oil Transfer to your Ninja Foodie's insert, and place the insert in your Foodi Lock Air Crisping lid and cook for 4 minutes at 390 degrees F Half through, make sure to give them a nice flip and keep cooking. Serve warm and enjoy!

Garlic And Lemon Prawn Delight
INGREDIENTS (4 Servings)

2 tablespoons olive oil
1 pound prawns
2 tablespoons garlic, minced
2/3 cup fish stock
1 tablespoon butter
2 tablespoons lemon juice
1 tablespoon lemon zest
Salt and pepper to taste

DIRECTIONS (PREP + COOK TIME: 10 MINUTES)
Set your Ninja Foodi to Saute mode and add butter and oil, let it heat up Stir in remaining ingredients. Lock lid and cook on LOW pressure for 5 minutes Quick release pressure. Serve and enjoy

Lovely Panko Cod

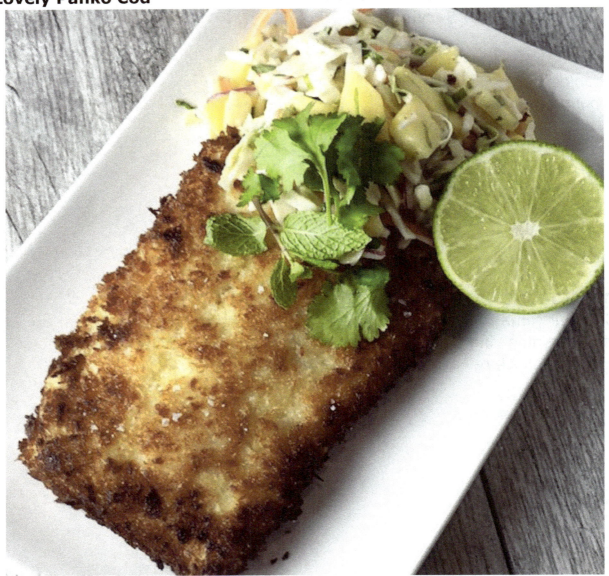

INGREDIENTS (6 Servings)

2 uncooked cod fillets,
6 ounces each
3 teaspoons kosher salt
¾ cup panko bread crumbs
2 tablespoons butter, melted
 ¼ cup fresh parsley, minced
1 lemon.

Zested and juiced

DIRECTIONS (PREP + COOK TIME: 20 MINUTES)

Pre-heat your Ninja Foodi at 390 degrees F and place Air Crisper basket inside Season cod and salt Take a bowl and add bread crumbs, parsley, lemon juice, zest, butter, and mix well Coat fillets with the bread crumbs mixture and place fillets in your Air Crisping basket Lock Air Crisping lid and cook on Air Crisp mode for 15 minutes at 360 degrees F Serve and enjoy!

Ranch Warm Fillets
INGREDIENTS (4 Servings)

¼ cup panko
½ packet ranch dressing mix powder
 1 and ¼ tablespoons vegetable oil
1 egg beaten
2 tilapia fillets
A garnish of herbs and chilies

DIRECTIONS (PREP + COOK TIME: 18 MINUTES)

Pre-heat your Ninja Foodi with the Crisping Basket inside at 350 degrees F Take a bowl and mix in ranch dressing and panko Beat eggs in a shallow bowl and keep it on the side Dip fillets in the eggs, then in the panko mix Place fillets in your Ninja Foodie's insert and transfer insert to Ninja Foodi Lock Air Crisping Lid and Air Crisp for 13 minutes at 350 degrees F Garnish with chilies and herbs. Enjoy!

Breathtaking Cod Fillets
INGREDIENTS (4 Servings)

1 pound frozen cod fish fillets
2 garlic cloves, halved
1 cup chicken broth
½ cup packed parsley
2 tablespoons oregano
2 tablespoons almonds, sliced
½ teaspoon paprika

DIRECTIONS (PREP + COOK TIME: 20 MINUTES)

Take the fish out of the freezer and let it defrost Take a food processor and stir in garlic, oregano, parsley, paprika, 1 tablespoon almond and process. Set your Ninja Foodi to "SAUTE" mode and add olive oil, let it heat up Add remaining almonds and toast, transfer to a towel. Pour broth in a pot and add herb mixture Cut fish into 4 pieces and place in a steamer basket, transfer steamer basket to the pot Lock lid and cook on HIGH pressure for 3 minutes. Quick release pressure once has done Serve steamed fish by pouring over the sauce.Enjoy!

Spiced Up Cajun Style Tilapia
INGREDIENTS (4 Servings)

4 tilapia fillets,
6 ounces each
1 cup ghee
2 teaspoons cayenne pepper
2 tablespoons smoked paprika
2 teaspoons garlic powder
2 teaspoons onion powder
Pinch of salt
1 teaspoon dried oregano
1 teaspoon dried thyme
1 cup of water

DIRECTIONS (PREP + COOK TIME: 15 MINUTES)
Take a small bowl and add cayenne pepper, smoked paprika, garlic powder, onion powder, salt, pepper, dried oregano, dried thyme and ghee Dip the fillets into the seasoned ghee mix. Add 1 cup of water to your Ninja Foodi Place steamer rack and place the fillets on the rack Lock lid and cook on HIGH pressure for 5 minutes. Release naturally over 10 minutes Transfer to serving platter and garnish with parsley. Serve and enjoy!

Orange Sauce And Salmon
INGREDIENTS (4 Servings)

1 pound salmon
1 tablespoon coconut amino
2 teaspoons ginger, minced
1 teaspoon garlic, minced
1 teaspoon salt
2 tablespoons sugar marmalade

DIRECTIONS (PREP + COOK TIME: 45 MINUTES)

Take a zip bag and add the Salmon. Take a bowl and add all of the ingredients and mix well Pour the mixture into the salmon container bag and mix well to ensure that the salmon is coated well. Allow it to marinate for 30 minutes Add 2 cups of water to the Ninja Foodi. Carefully put a steamer rack/trivet on top of your Foodi Add the marinated salmon and sauce on the rack Lock up the lid and cook on LOW pressure for 3 minutes Allow the pressure to release naturally.Serve or broil for 3-4 minutes for a brown texture Alternatively, you may bake the salmon at 350 degrees Fahrenheit for a slightly flaky fish. Enjoy!

Favorite Salmon Stew
INGREDIENTS (4 Servings)

1 cup fish broth
Salt and pepper to taste
1 medium onion, chopped
 1-2 pounds salmon fillets, cubed
1 tablespoon butter

DIRECTIONS (PREP + COOK TIME: 16 MINUTES) Add the listed ingredients to a large-sized bowl and let the shrimp marinate for 30-60 minutes Grease the inner pot of the Ninja Foodi with butter and transfer marinated shrimp to the pot Lock the lid and select "Bake/Roast" mode and bake for 15 minutes at 355 degrees F Once done, serve and enjoy!

Asian Salmon And Veggie Meal

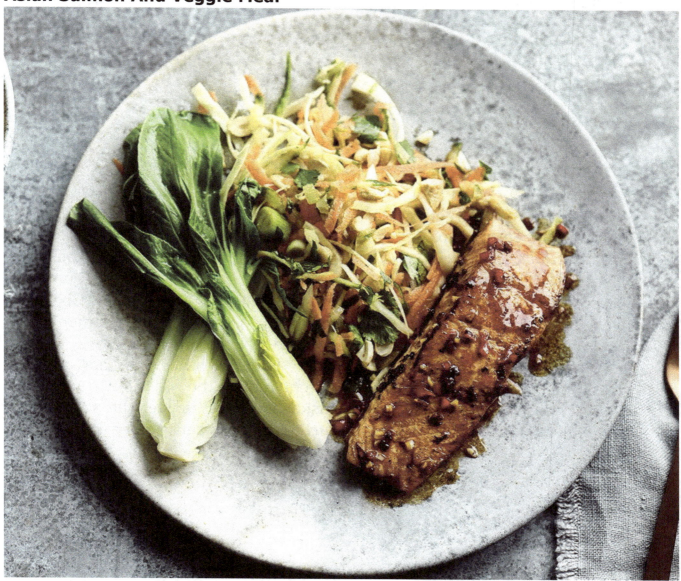

INGREDIENTS (4 Servings)

For Fish 2 medium salmon fillets
1 garlic cloves, diced
2 teaspoons ginger, grated
¼ a long red chili, diced
Salt as needed
2 tablespoons coconut aminos
1 teaspoon agave nectar For Veggies
½ pound mixed green veggies

1 large carrot, sliced
1 garlic clove, diced
½ lime, juice
1 tablespoon tamari sauce
1 tablespoon olive oil
½ teaspoon sesame oil

DIRECTIONS (PREP + COOK TIME: 2 hours and 5 MINUTES) Add 1 cup of water to your Ninja Foodi and place a trivet inside Place fish fillets inside a heatproof tin (small enough to fit inside the pot) and sprinkle diced garlic, chili, and ginger on top. Season with salt and pepper Take a small bowl and create a mixture of tamari and agave nectar Pour the mixture over the fillets. Place tin with salmon on top of the trivet Lock up the lid and cook on HIGH pressure for 3 minutes and perform a quick release Cut the vegetables and place the veggies in a steam basket. Sprinkle garlic Place the steamer basket with veggies on top of the salmon tin and drizzle lime juice, olive oil, tamari, sesame oil. Season with salt and pepper Lock up the lid and cook on HIGH pressure for 0 minutes (just the time required for the pressure to build up). Quick release the remove the and basket and tin Transfer the salmon to a plate alongside veggies and pour any remaining sauce over the salmon, enjoy!

Great Seafood Stew
INGREDIENTS (4 Servings)

3 tablespoons extra virgin olive oil
2 bay leaves
2 teaspoons paprika
1 small onion, sliced
1 small green bell pepper
2 garlic cloves, mashed
Salt and pepper to taste
1 cup fish stock
1 and ½ pound meat fish
1 pound shrimp, cleaned and deveined
12 neck clams ¼ cup cilantro, garnish
1 tablespoon extra virgin olive oil

DIRECTIONS (PREP + COOK TIME: 20 MINUTES) Set your Ninja Foodi to Saute mode and add olive oil Add bay leaves and paprika and Saute for 30 seconds Add onion, bell pepper, tomatoes, 2 tablespoons of cilantro, garlic and season with salt and pepper. Stir for a few minutes . Add fish stock Season fish with salt and pepper and Nestle the clams and shrimp among the veggies in the Ninja Foodi. Add fish on top Lock up the lid and cook on HIGH pressure for 10 minutes Release the pressure over 10 minutes Divide the stew amongst bowls and drizzle 1 tablespoon of olive oil Sprinkle 2 tablespoon of cilantro and serve. Enjoy!

Juicy Mediterranean Cod
INGREDIENTS (4 Servings)

6 Fresh Cod
 3 tablespoons clarified butter
1 lemon, juiced
1 onion, sliced
1 teaspoon salt
½ teaspoon pepper
1 teaspoon oregano
1 can (28 ounces) tomatoes, diced

DIRECTIONS (PREP + COOK TIME: 20 MINUTES)
Set your pot to Saute mode and add clarified butter Once the butter is hot, add the rest of the ingredients and stir (except fish).Saute for 10 minutes Arrange the fish portions in the sauce and spoon the sauce over the fish to coat it Lock up the lid and cook under HIGH pressure for 5 minutes. Perform a quick release and serve!

Delicious Smoked Salmon And Spinach Frittata
INGREDIENTS (4 Servings)

10 whole eggs
¼ cup unsweetened almond milk
1 teaspoon garlic powder
1 teaspoon orange-chili-garlic sauce
 ½ teaspoon of sea salt
¼ teaspoon freshly ground black pepper
8 ounces smoked salmon, flaked
8 ounces shiitake mushrooms, sliced
2 cups baby spinach Oil for greasing

DIRECTIONS (PREP + COOK TIME: 8 hours and 10 MINUTES)
Take a large sized bowl and add eggs, orange chili garlic sauce, almond milk, garlic powder and season with salt and pepper. Fold in smoked salmon, spinach and mushrooms Mix well. Grease Ninja Foodi with oil. Pour egg mix in Ninja Foodi Close lid and cook on SLOW COOK Mode (LOW) for 8 hours. Serve and enjoy! Dijon Flavored Lemon Whitefish (Prepping time: 5 minutes\ Cooking time: 2 minutes |For 4 servings) Ingredients 1 pound whitefish fillets 2 tablespoons Dijon mustard 1 teaspoon horseradish, grated 1 tablespoon fresh lemon juice 1 teaspoon fresh ginger, grated ½ teaspoon salt and black pepper (each) 1 lemon, sliced ½ tablespoon olive oil 1 cup of water Directions Mix in Dijon mustard, lemon juice and horseradish in a bowl Season white fish fillets with salt and pepper, add Dijon marinade Let it marinate for 20 minutes. Add water to your Ninja Foodi and place a steamer rack inside Put fillets on the rack and pour marinade on top Lock lid and cook on HIGH pressure for 20 minutes Release pressure naturally over 10 minutes. Enjoy!

Very Low Carb Clam Chowder
INGREDIENTS (4 Servings)

13 slices bacon, thick cut
2 cups chicken broth
1 cup celery, chopped
1 cup onion, chopped
 6 cups baby clams, with juice
2 cups heavy whipping cream
1 teaspoon salt
1 teaspoon ground thyme
1 teaspoon pepper

DIRECTIONS (PREP + COOK TIME: 4 hours and 25 MINUTES)
Take a skillet and place it over medium heat, cook bacon until crispy Drain and crumble the bacon. Chop onion, celery and add them to the pan Once tender add veggies alongside remaining ingredients to your Ninja Foodi Lock lid and cook on SLOW COOK MODE(LOW) for 4-6 hours. Serve and enjoy!

Indian Fish Curry
INGREDIENTS (4 Servings)

 2 tablespoons of coconut oil
10 curry leaves
1 cup of onion, chopped
A tablespoon of ginger
1 tablespoon of garlic
1/2 jalapeno or Serrano chili pepper, sliced
1 cup of tomatoes, chopped
A teaspoon of ground coriander
1/4 teaspoon of ground cumin
1/2 teaspoon of turmeric
1/2 teaspoon of black pepper
1 teaspoon of salt
2 tablespoons of water
1 cup (1/2 of 14 oz can) of canned coconut milk
1 1/2 lbs of fish fillets, cut into 2-inches pieces
1 teaspoon of lime juice

DIRECTIONS (PREP + COOK TIME: 15 MINUTES) Warm up the coconut oil on sauté mode. Add the curry leaves and stir for some seconds. Add the onions, garlic, ginger, and green chilies. Continue cooking until the onions are soft. Add the tomatoes and sauté them until it starts to break. Add cumin, coriander, turmeric, salt, and black pepper. Sauté for some seconds until it starts to burn. Add water to deglaze and add the coconut milk. Insert a reversible rack in the Foodi and put the fish cutlets in it. Close the pressure lid and steam the fish for 2 minutes. Quick release the accumulated vapor and open the lid. Remove the rack containing fish and add lime juice to the curry mixture. Stir. Transfer fish and its gravy into bowl and garnish with fresh tomato slices and chopped cilantro.

Garlicky Shrimp Scampi

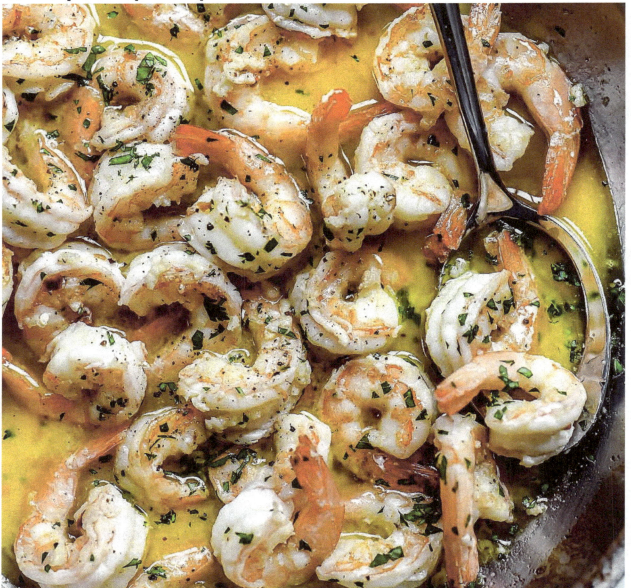

INGREDIENTS (4 Servings)

1 1/4 pounds of shrimp (peeled and de-veined)
4 tablespoons of butter
3 cloves of garlic, chopped roughly
1/4 cup of chardonnay wine
1/4 cup of lemon juice
1/4 teaspoon of red pepper flakes
1/4 cup of chopped parsley

2 scallions (white and light green part), sliced
1/2 cup of Parmesan cheese, shredded
Salt and black pepper

DIRECTIONS (PREP + COOK TIME: 25 MINUTES) Preheat your Foodi by sautéing it over medium high. Add butter to the pot followed by the chopped garlic. Let it cook until the garlic softens. Stir. Add the de-veined shrimp and red pepper flakes. Add the lemon juice and wine. Close the pressure lid and cook the shrimp on high mode for 10 minutes. Quick release the accumulated steam and open the lid. Add the chopped parsley and scallions. Stir. Season the mixture with salt and pepper Serve while topped with Parmesan cheese, if desired.

Brazilian Fish Stew
INGREDIENTS (5 Servings)

For the Stew:
1 red bell pepper, sliced
1 onion, diced
5 garlic cloves, minced
8 oz of fish broth
14 oz of canned tomatoes, crushed
6 oz of full-fat coconut milk, canned
1 tablespoon of ground cumin
2 tablespoons of coconut oil
1 tablespoon of smoked paprika
1/2 teaspoon of black pepper
A teaspoon of salt
¼ and ½ teaspoons of ground cayenne
Finishing:
1 1/2 pounds of cod or halibut
A tablespoon of lime juice
2 tablespoons of coconut oil
1 tablespoon of fresh cilantro or parsley, chopped

DIRECTIONS (PREP + COOK TIME: 35 MINUTES) Combine all the ingredients in your Foodi and stir. Seal the pressure lid and cook on high mode for 10 minutes. When the cooking time elapses, quick release the accumulated steam. Open the lid and set the Foodi to sauté mode. Thicken the stew over medium heat for around 10 minutes, while stirring frequently. Meanwhile, prepare the fish by removing its skin and bones and then pat drying it with paper towels. Cut the fish into one inch pieces. Once stew has thickened, add the fish cutlets and stir. Cook for 5 minutes and turn off the sauté function. Add the coconut oil and lime juice. Stir. Serve while topped with chopped parsley or cilantro.

Hot Prawns with Cocktail Sauce
INGREDIENTS (4 Servings)

1 teaspoon of chili powder
½ teaspoon of sea salt
1 teaspoon of chili flakes
½ teaspoon of fresh ground black pepper
8 fresh king prawns
1 tablespoon of ketchup
3 tablespoons of mayonnaise
1 tablespoons of wine

DIRECTIONS (PREP + COOK TIME: 16 MINUTES) Preheat the Foodi unit on air crisp mode at 300°F. Combine all spices in a bowl. Add the prawns and toss with the spices to coat. Put the prawns in the basket and cook crisp for 6 minutes. Combine the sauce ingredients in a bowl. Serve the hot spicy prawns with the sauce.

Catfish with French Sauce
INGREDIENTS (4 Servings)

1½ pounds of catfish fillets (rinse, pat-dry, and cut)
1 (14½-ounce) can of diced tomatoes
2 teaspoons of dried minced onion
¼ teaspoon of onion powder
1 teaspoon of dried minced garlic
¼ teaspoon of garlic powder
1 teaspoon of hot paprika
1 medium green bell pepper (seeded and diced)
¼ teaspoon of dried tarragon
1 celery stalk, diced finely
Salt and freshly ground pepper
½ cup of chili sauce
¼ teaspoon of sugar

DIRECTIONS (PREP + COOK TIME: 15 MINUTES) Add all the ingredients (except the fish fillets) to the pot and mix thoroughly. Add the fillets and stir. Close the pressure lid and cook the fillets mixture on low mode for five minutes. Quick release the accumulated pressure and open the lid. Stir gently and add more seasonings, if required.

Shrimp with Tomatoes and Feta
INGREDIENTS (6 Servings)

2 tablespoons of butter
1/2 teaspoon of red pepper flakes
A tablespoon of garlic
11/2 cups of onions, chopped
A (14.5oz) canned tomatoes
1 teaspoon of salt
1 teaspoon of dried oregano
1 lb of frozen shrimp, shelled
For serving:
1 cup of crumbled feta cheese
1/2 cup of black olives, sliced
1/4 cup of parsley, chopped

DIRECTIONS (PREP + COOK TIME: 22 MINUTES) Set your Foodi to sauté mode. Add butter to melt. Add garlic, red pepper flakes, tomatoes, onions, salt, and oregano.   Add the frozen shrimps and close the pressure lid. Cook the shrimp mixture on low mode for one minute. Quick release the in-built pressure and open the lid. Cool and serve it sprinkled with feta cheese, sliced olives, and chopped parsley. Enjoy your tomato shrimp with cauliflower rice or as dipping for buttered French bread.

Red Snapper with miso
INGREDIENTS (4 Servings)

2 pounds of red snapper fillets
1 tablespoon of red miso paste
A tablespoon of rice wine
1 (2-inch) fresh ginger, peeled and cut long
4 green onions (halved lengthwise and cut into 2"pieces)
2 teaspoons of sesame oil
A teaspoon of dark soy sauce
2 teaspoons of fermented black beans
2 garlic cloves (peeled and minced)
½ teaspoon of Asian chili paste
Salt Water

DIRECTIONS (PREP + COOK TIME: 24 MINUTES) Insert a rack in the Foodi. Pour some water into the pot. Mix miso with rice wine, black beans, sesame oil, chili paste, and soy sauce in a bowl. Sprinkle salt over the mixture and rub the snapper fillets with it. Put half of the peeled ginger on the pan. Add half of the garlic. Pour half of the green onions over the garlic and ginger. Place the fillets in the pan and sprinkle them with the ginger mixture. Transfer them to the fitted rack. Close the pressure lid and cook on low mode for 3 minutes. Quick release the accumulated steam and serve.

Calamari with Tomato Stew

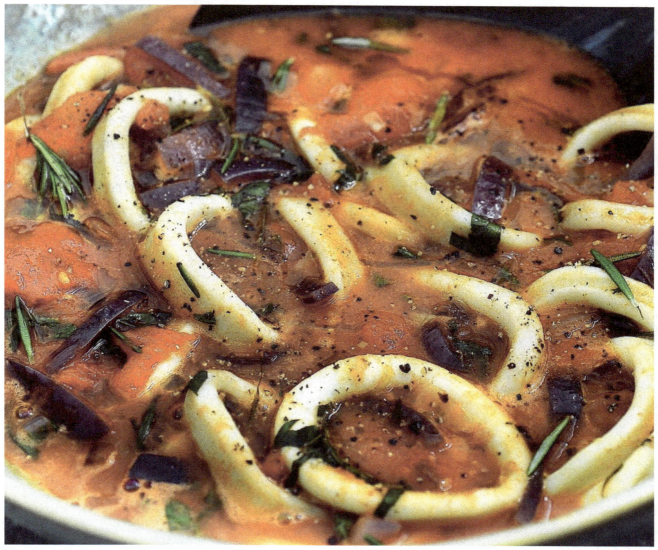

INGREDIENTS (4 Servings)

2½ pounds of calamari
2 tablespoons of essential olive oil
1 small white onion (peeled and diced)
1 small stalk celery, finely diced
1 small carrot (peeled and grated)
3 cloves garlic (peeled and minced)
1 can (28-oz) of diced tomatoes
Salt and freshly ground black pepper
½ cup of white wine

1/3 of cup water
1 tablespoon of fresh parsley
A tablespoon of fresh basil

DIRECTIONS (PREP + COOK TIME: 25 MINUTES) Sauté the celery stalk and carrots in oil for two minutes. Add onions and cook for 3 minutes. Add the garlic and cook for thirty seconds. Clean and pat-dry the calamari and add it to the Foodi. Add the remaining ingredients and close the pressure lid. Cook the mixture on low mode for 10 minutes and quick release the in-built steam. Open the lid and add the fresh herbs. Serve your calamari dish hot.

Fish Steaks with Olive Sauce and Tomato
INGREDIENTS (2 Servings)

2 firm fish steaks (cut thickly into ½ inches)
2/3 cup of sliced mushrooms
2 tablespoons of extra virgin olive oil
1/2 cup of chopped onion
2 garlic cloves, minced
4 Roma tomatoes, chopped
2 tablespoons of capers, drained
1/4 cup of chopped and pitted kalamata olives
2 tablespoons of fresh parsley, minced
1/8 teaspoon of crushed red pepper, dried
1/4 cup of white wine
1/4 teaspoon of salt

DIRECTIONS (PREP + COOK TIME: 24 MINUTES) Preheat the Foodi unit on sauté mode. Add garlic and onion in oil and cook for3 minutes. Add the remaining ingredients (except the fish) and stir. Put the fish steaks in the basket and insert it in the Foodi. Close the pressure lid and steam the fish for five minutes. Enjoy!

Buttered Salmon
INGREDIENTS (2 Servings)

2 (6-ounce) salmon fillets
Salt and ground black pepper, as required
1 tablespoon butter, melted

DIRECTIONS (Prep + Cook Time: 20 minutes)
Arrange the greased "Cook & Crisp Basket" in the pot of Ninja Foodi. Close the Ninja Foodi with crisping lid and select "Air Crisp". Set the temperature to 360 degrees F for 5 minutes. Press "Start/Stop" to begin preheating. Season each salmon fillet with salt and black pepper and then coat with the melted butter. After preheating, open the lid. Arrange the salmon fillets into the prepared"Cook & Crisp Basket" in a single layer. Close the Ninja Foodi with crisping lid and select "Air Crisp". Set the temperature to 360 degrees F for 10 minutes. Press "Start/Stop" to begin cooking. Open the lid and serve hot.

Parmesan Tilapia
INGREDIENTS (4 Servings)

½ cup Parmesan cheese, grated
¼ cup mayonnaise
¼ cup fresh lemon juice
Salt and ground black pepper, as required
4 (4-ounce) tilapia fillets
2 tablespoons fresh cilantro, chopped

DIRECTIONS (Prep + Cook Time: 4 hours 10 minutes)
In a bowl, mix together all ingredients except tilapia fillets and cilantro. Coat the fillets with mayonnaise mixture evenly. Place the filets over a large piece of foil. Wrap the foil around fillets to seal them. Arrange the foil packet in the bottom of Ninja Foodi. Close the Ninja Foodi with crisping lid and select "Slow Cooker". Set on "Low" for 3-4 hours. Press "Start/Stop" to begin

cooking.   Open the lid and transfer the foil parcel onto a platter. Carefully open the parcel and serve hot with the garnishing of cilantro.

Glazed Haddock
INGREDIENTS (4 Servings)

1 garlic clove, minced
¼ teaspoon fresh ginger, grated finely
½ cup low-sodium soy sauce
¼ cup fresh lime juice
½ cup chicken broth
¼ cup sugar
¼ teaspoon red pepper flakes, crushed
1 pound haddock steak

DIRECTIONS (Prep + Cook Time: 26 minutes)
Select"Sauté/Sear" setting of Ninja Foodi and place all ingredients except haddock steak. Press "Start/Stop" to begin and cook for about 3-4 minutes, stirring continuously. Press "Start/Stop" to stop cooking and transfer the mixture into a bowl. Set aside to cool. In a bowl, reserve half of the marinade. In a resealable bag, add the remaining marinade and haddock steak. Seal the bag and shake to coat well. Refrigerate for about 30 minutes. Arrange the greased "Cook & Crisp Basket" in the pot of Ninja Foodi. Close the Ninja Foodi with crisping lid and select "Air Crisp". Set the temperature to 390 degrees F for 5 minutes. Press "Start/Stop" to begin preheating. After preheating, open the lid. Place the haddock steak into the "Cook & Crisp Basket". Close the Ninja Foodi with crisping lid and select "Air Crisp". Set the temperature to 390 degrees F for 11 minutes. Press "Start/Stop" to begin cooking. Open the lid and transfer the haddock steak onto a serving platter. Immediately coat the haddock steaks with the remaining glaze. Serve immediately.

Shrimp Scampi
INGREDIENTS (3 Servings)

4 tablespoons salted butter
1 tablespoon fresh lemon juice
1 tablespoon garlic, minced
2 teaspoons red pepper flakes, crushed
1 pound shrimp, peeled and deveined
2 tablespoons fresh basil, chopped
1 tablespoon fresh chives, chopped
2 tablespoons chicken broth

DIRECTIONS (Prep + Cook Time: 22 minutes)
Arrange a 7-inch round baking pan in the "Cook & Crisp Basket". Now, arrange the "Cook & Crisp Basket" in the pot of Ninja Foodi. Close the Ninja Foodi with crisping lid and select "Air Crisp". Set the temperature to 325 degrees F for 5 minutes. Press "Start/Stop" to begin preheating. After preheating, open the lid and carefully remove the pan from Ninja Foodi. In the heated pan, place butter, lemon juice, garlic, and red pepper flakes and mix well. Place the pan in the "Cook & Crisp Basket". Close the Ninja Foodi with crisping lid and select "Air Crisp". Set the temperature to 325 degrees F for 7 minutes. Press "Start/Stop" to begin cooking. After 2 minutes of cooking, stir in the shrimp, basil, chives and broth. Open the lid and place the pan onto a wire rack for about 1 minute. Stir the mixture and serve hot.

Seafood & Tomato Stew

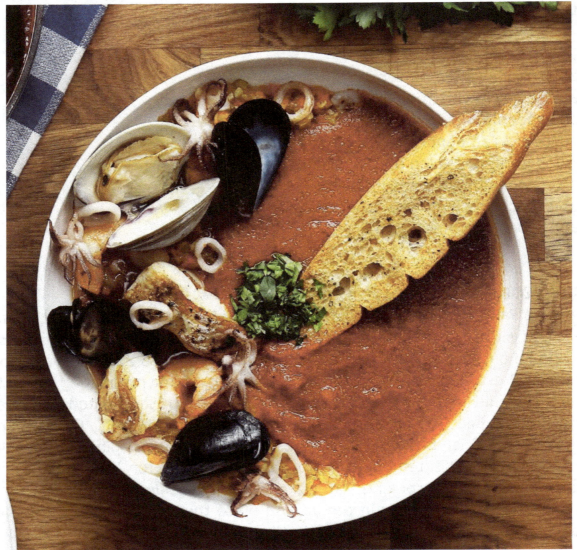

INGREDIENTS (8 Servings)

2 tablespoons olive oil
1 pound tomatoes, chopped
1 large yellow onion, chopped finely
2 garlic cloves, minced
2 teaspoons curry powder
6 sprigs fresh parsley
Salt and ground black pepper, as required
1½ cups chicken broth
1½ pounds salmon, cut into cubes

1½ pounds shrimp, peeled and deveined

DIRECTIONS (Prep + Cook Time: 5 hours)

In the pot of Ninja Foodi, add all ingredients except seafood and mix well. Close the Ninja Foodi with crisping lid and select "Slow Cooker". Set on "High" for 4 hours. Press "Start/Stop" to begin cooking. Open the lid and stir in the seafood. Now, set on "Low" for 50 minutes. Press "Start/Stop" to begin cooking. Open the lid and serve hot.

Shrimp Chicken Jambalaya
INGREDIENTS (4-6 Servings)

12 ounces of large shrimp (peeled and deveined)
2 skinless and boneless chicken (halved and cubed)
1 cup of rice, uncooked
1 large green pepper, diced
1 onion, chopped
3 stalks celery, sliced
2 garlic cloves, minced
1 tablespoon of vegetable oil
1 can (8 oz) of tomato sauce
1-1/4 cups of chicken broth
1/2 teaspoon of dried thyme leaves
1/2 teaspoon of salt 1 bay leaf
1/2 teaspoon of white pepper
2 dashes of hot pepper sauce
1/4 teaspoon of red pepper cayenne
1/2 teaspoon of sage

DIRECTIONS (PREP + COOK TIME: 25 MINUTES) Preheat the Foodi unit for 5 minutes. Sauté the onion, chicken, garlic green pepper, and celery until they tenderizes. Add the remaining ingredients and close the pressure lid. Cook the mixture on high mode for 9 minutes. Quick release the accumulated pressure.

Mussels and Chorizo
INGREDIENTS (4 Servings)

A small French baguette, ½" slices
2 tablespoons of organic olive oil
2 tablespoons of butter
2 shallots (peeled and thinly sliced)
2 garlic cloves (peeled and thinly sliced)
1 cup of fennel, sliced thinly
A (6 oz) Spanish-style chorizo (casings off and cut into ¼" pieces)
1 cup of diced tomatoes
1/4 cup of heavy cream
3/4 cup of white wine
2 pounds of mussels, cleaned and de-bearded
2 tablespoons of fresh parsley, chopped
Juice from a lemon

DIRECTIONS (PREP + COOK TIME: 30 MINUTES) Brush the baguette slices with a little organic olive oil. Insert the reversible rack in the pot and put the brushed slices in it. Close the crisping lid and toast the baguette at 400°F for 5 minutes. Once cooked, remove the rack with toasted baguette and set it aside. Preheat the multi-cooker in sauté mode and then add butter, garlic, shallots, and fennel. Sauté the spices for 2 minutes. Add tomatoes, chorizo, heavy cream, wine, and mussels. Seal the pressure lid and cook on low mode for 3 minutes. Quick release the pressure and transfer the mussels with into a platter. Sprinkle them with lemon juice and parsley. Serve with toast.

Creamy Crab
INGREDIENTS (4 Servings)

1 pound of lump crabmeat (raw)
½ cup of heavy cream
4 tablespoons of butter
¼ cup of chicken broth
½ stalk celery, diced finely
1 small red onion (peeled and finely diced)
Salt and freshly ground black pepper

DIRECTIONS (PREP + COOK TIME: 24 MINUTES) Preheat the unit on Sauté mode for a minute. Add butter and let it melt. Add the celery and cook until it softens. Stir. Add the onions and cook for 3 minutes. Add the chicken broth and crabmeat. Stir and close the pressure lid. Cook on low mode for 3 minutes. Quick release the accumulated pressure and open the lid. Add cream and mix. Add salt and pepper. Stir and set aside. Melt butter over medium heat. Add celery and sauté until it softens. Add the onion and stir. Sauté the mixture for 3 minutes. Add the crabmeat and broth. Stir and secure the lid. Cook them on low mode for 3 minutes and quick release open the lid. Stir. Add the heavy cream followed by salt and pepper. Enjoy.

Paella
INGREDIENTS (4-6 Servings)

2 tablespoons of extra virgin olive oil
3 links of chorizo, sliced
3 boneless skinless chicken thighs (cut)
1 medium onion (peeled and chopped finely)
2 cloves of garlic (peeled and minced)
 1 small red bell pepper, chopped
A teaspoon of paprika
1/2 teaspoon of oregano, dried
1/4 teaspoon of crushed red pepper
1/2 teaspoon of pepper
A teaspoon of kosher salt
Pinch of saffron threads, crumbled
A can (14 oz) of diced tomatoes
1/2 cup of chicken stock
1/4 cup of white wine
A cup of basmati rice
1 pound of mussels (scrubbed and de-bearded)
1 bag (12 oz) of frozen jumbo shrimp (peeled and deveined)
Juice from one lemon
2 tablespoons of fresh parsley, for garnishing

DIRECTIONS (PREP + COOK TIME: 27 MINUTES) Preheat your Foodi on sauté mode for a minute. Add the chicken thighs and sliced chorizos in oil. Cook for 5 minutes. Add the onions, garlic, red pepper, and spices. Sauté for another 5 minutes. Add the wine, stock, rice, tomatoes, shrimp, and mussels. Stir. Close the pressure lid and cook for 2 minutes. Quick release the accumulated pressure and open the lid. Transfer your Paella into a large bowl. Serve while topped with parsley and fresh lemon juice.

Seared Shrimp and Rice with Fruity
INGREDIENTS (4 Servings)

A cup of basmati rice
1 cup of water
1 1/2 teaspoons of sea salt, divided
3 tablespoons of canola oil
3 tablespoons of fresh lime juice, divided
1 lb (31-35) of large shrimp, uncooked
1 1/2 teaspoons of crab seasoning
A teaspoon of garlic powder
1 teaspoon of smoked paprika
1/2 teaspoon of onion powder
1 mango (peeled and chopped)
1/2 teaspoon of sugar
1/4 cup of red onion (peeled and chopped)
1 small bell pepper (red,) chopped
1/2 cup of pineapple, chopped
3 scallions, finely sliced 1 avocado, sliced

DIRECTIONS (PREP + COOK TIME: 30 MINUTES) Peel the shrimp, devein it and remove its tail. Put it aside. If frozen, thaw it first. Add, water, rice, and a teaspoon of salt in the Foodi. Close the pressure lid and cook on high mode for 2 minutes. Quick release the in-built pressure and open the lid. Meanwhile, toss the shrimp with the crab seasoning, onion powder, garlic powder, sugar, smoked paprika, and 2 tablespoons of oil. Open the pressure lid and add the remaining oil and a teaspoon of lime juice. Stir. Fix the rack in the rice-pot. Place shrimp on the rack and close the crisping lid. Broil it for 7 minutes. Halfway, open the lid and flip the shrimp. Meanwhile, add the mango, pineapple, bell pepper, red onion, the remaining salt and the lime juice. After the cooking time elapses, serve the broiled shrimp with rice. Top with avocado slices, scallions, and salsa.

Garlic Shrimp with Risotto Primavera

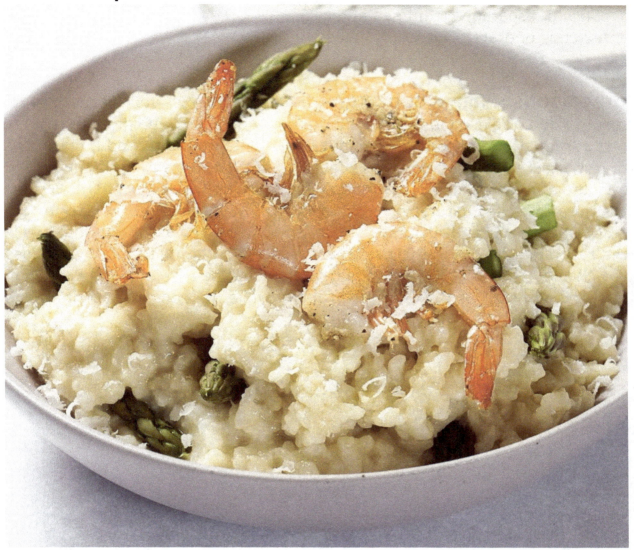

INGREDIENTS (4 Servings)

2 tablespoons of organic olive oil, divided
1 small onion (peeled and diced finely)
4 cloves garlic (peeled, minced, and divided)
3 teaspoons of sea salt, divided
5 1/2 cups of chicken stock
2 glasses of short- grained rice
16 uncooked jumbo shrimp (peeled and deveined)
2 teaspoons of garlic powder
1 teaspoon of ground black pepper

2 tablespoons of butter Juice from a lemon
1 bunch of asparagus (trimmed and cut)
1 1/2 cups of grated Parmesan cheese

DIRECTIONS (PREP + COOK TIME: 39 MINUTES) Set your Foodi to sauté mode. Add a tablespoon of oil. Add the onion and cook until it softens. Add half of the garlic and cook for 1 minute or until its fragrant. Add 2 teaspoons of salt, stock, and rice. Close the pressure lid. Toss the shrimp in the oil and add the remaining garlic, garlic powder, salt, and black pepper. Let the pressure release naturally for 10 minutes before quick releasing the rest. Open the lid and add butter, fresh lemon juice, and asparagus into it. Fix the reversible rack over the risotto and add the shrimp into the rack. Close the crisping lid and broil for 8 minutes. Remove the rack and add Parmesan into the risotto. Stir. Serve your meal while topped with shrimp and Parmesan.

Salmon with Orange Ginger Sauce
INGREDIENTS (4 Servings)

1 pound of salmon
2 teaspoons of minced ginger
1 tablespoon of dark soy sauce
1 teaspoon of garlic, minced
½ teaspoon of salt
1-11/2 teaspoon of ground pepper
2 tablespoons of marmalade, low sugar

DIRECTIONS (PREP + COOK TIME: 30 MINUTES) Put salmon in a Ziploc bag. Add the minced ginger, dark soy sauce, garlic, marmalade, salt, and pepper. Let it marinate for 30 minutes. Add 2 glasses of water in the Foodi. Fix a reversible rack over it and add the seasoned salmon with sauce. Close the pressure lid and cook on low mode for 3 minutes. Allow the in-built pressure to escape naturally. Close the crisping lid and broil the contents for 3 minutes. Alternatively, bake the seasoned fish at a temperature of 350°F for 5 minutes.

Thai Shrimp Soup Lime,
INGREDIENTS (6 Servings)

2 tablespoons of unsalted butter, divided
½ lb of medium shrimp (uncooked, peeled, and deveined)
½ yellow onion, diced
2 cloves of garlic, minced
2 tablespoons of fish sauce
4 servings of chicken broth
2 tablespoons of lime juice
1 tablespoon of coconut aminos or tamari sauce
2½ teaspoons of red curry paste
1 stalk of lemongrass (bruised and chopped)
1 cup of fresh white mushrooms, sliced
1 tablespoon of fresh cinnamon, grated
½ teaspoon of freshly ground black pepper
1 teaspoon of sea salt
1 can(13.66-oz) of unsweetened, full-fat coconut milk
3 tablespoons of fresh cilantro, chopped

DIRECTIONS (PREP + COOK TIME: 11 MINUTES) Set your Foodi to sauté mode. Add a tablespoon of butter and allow it to melt. Add the shrimp and stir until it turns pink. Transfer it into a bowl and set aside. Add the remaining butter into the pot and let it melt. Add onion and the garlic. Sauté for 3 minutes or until it turns translucent. Add the chicken broth, fish sauce, lime juice, tamari sauce or coconut aminos, red curry paste, grated cinnamon, mushrooms, lemongrass, sea salt, and black pepper. Mix well. Close the pressure lid and cook on high mode for 5 minutes. When cooking time elapses, let the pressure to escape naturally for 5 minutes. Quick release the remaining pressure and open the lid. Add the coconut shrimp and milk. Stir to combine. Boil the soup on sauté mode for around 5 minutes. Let the soup rest for two minutes before serving. Serve with cilantro toppings.

Wild Salmon Tagine
INGREDIENTS (4 Servings)

Spice Paste:
41/2 oz of coriander leaves and stems
4 cloves of garlic
Juice from a lemon
Orange zest (one orange)
1 lemon zest
A tablespoon of ground paprika
1 tablespoon of apple cider vinegar
1 red chili (seeded and stem off)
A tablespoon of ground cumin
1/4 teaspoon of red pepper cayenne
1/4 teaspoon of sea salt
Tagine:
4 frozen salmon fillets
4 tablespoon of extra virgin organic olive oil
1 red onion
10 oz of sweet potatoes (peeled and diced)
2 carrots, diced
14 oz of chopped tomatoes (tinned)
A cup of stock, vegetable or fish
1.5 oz of dried cherries
2 oz of pitted olives
2 oranges (peeled and chopped)

DIRECTIONS (PREP + COOK TIME: 24 MINUTES) Preheat the Foodi pot. Puree all the spice paste ingredients. Spread a tablespoon of the paste on the fish. Melt butter in the Foodi and add the red onion, carrots, sweet potatoes, and the remaining spice mix. Sauté and stir for 5 minutes. Add the stock, tinned tomatoes, oranges, olives, and dried cherries. Place the frozen fish on top and seal the pressure lid. Cook on high mode for 4 minutes. Quick release the in-built vapor and open the lid. Serve your wild salmon tagine garnished with fresh herbs (preferably parsley and mint leaves.)

Gentle And Simple Fish
INGREDIENTS (4 Servings)

3 cups fish stock
1 onion, diced
1 cup broccoli, chopped
2 cups celery stalks, chopped
1 and ½ cups cauliflower, diced
1 carrot, sliced
1 pound white fish fillets, chopped
1 cup heavy cream   1 bay leaf
2 tablespoons butter
¼ teaspoon pepper
½ teaspoon salt
¼ teaspoon garlic powder

DIRECTIONS (PREP + COOK TIME: 25 MINUTES)

Set your Ninja Foodi to Saute mode and add butter, let it melt Add onion and carrots, cook for 3 minutes. Stir in remaining ingredients Lock lid and cook on HIGH pressure for 4 minutes.Naturally, release pressure over 10 minutes Discard bay leaf . Serve and enjoy!

Awesome Cherry Tomato Mackerel

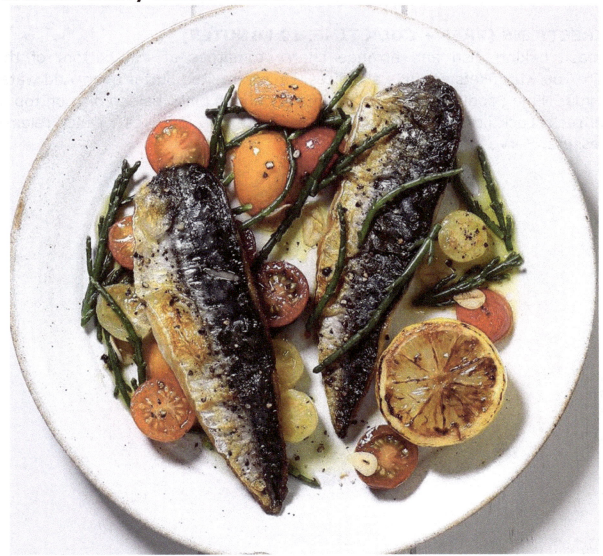

INGREDIENTS (4 Servings)

4 Mackerel fillets
¼ teaspoon onion powder
 ¼ teaspoon lemon powder
¼ teaspoon garlic powder
½ teaspoon salt
2 cups cherry tomatoes
3 tablespoons melted butter
1 and ½ cups of water
1 tablespoon black olives

DIRECTIONS (PREP + COOK TIME: 12 MINUTES)

Grease baking dish and arrange cherry tomatoes at the bottom of the dish Top with fillets sprinkle all spices. Drizzle melted butter over Add water to your Ninja Foodi Lower rack in Ninja Foodi and place baking dish on top of the rack Lock lid and cook on LOW pressure for 7 minutes . Quick release pressure. Serve and enjoy!

Delightful Salmon Fillets

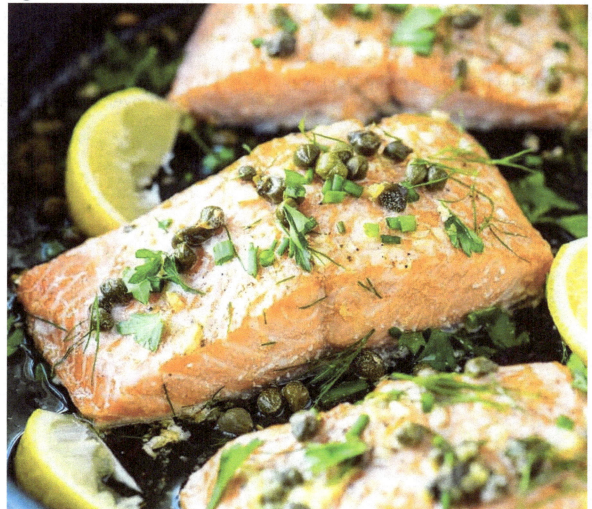

INGREDIENTS (4 Servings)

2 salmon fillets
¼ cup onion, chopped
2 stalks green onion stalks, chopped
1 whole egg
Almond meal as needed
Salt and pepper to taste
2 tablespoons olive oil

DIRECTIONS (PREP + COOK TIME: 10 MINUTES)

Add a cup of water to your Ninja Foodi and place a steamer rack on top Place the fish. Season the fish with salt and pepper and lock up the lid Cook on HIGH pressure for 3 minutes. Once done, quick release the pressure Remove the fish and allow it to cool Break the fillets into a bowl and add egg, yellow and green onions Add ½ a cup of almond meal and mix with your hand. Divide the mixture into patties Take a large skillet and place it over medium heat. Add oil and cook the patties.Enjoy!

Salmon in Dill Sauce

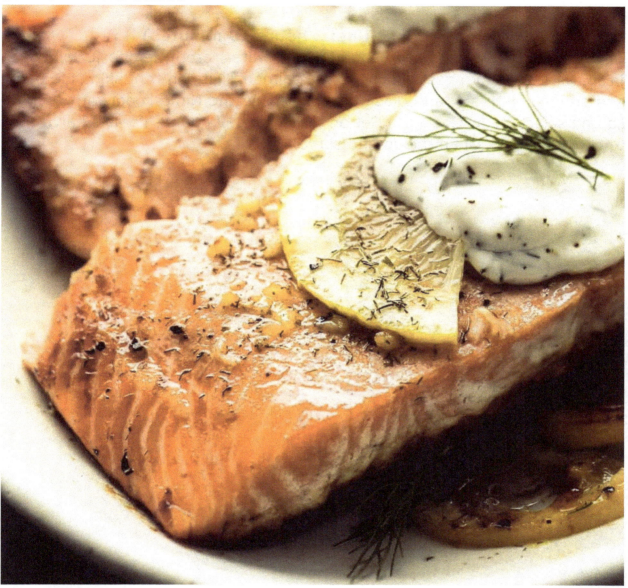

INGREDIENTS (6 Servings)

2 cups water
1 cup chicken broth
2 tablespoons fresh lemon juice
¼ cup fresh dill, chopped
½ teaspoon lemon zest, grated
6 (4-ounce) salmon fillets
Salt and ground black pepper, as required

DIRECTIONS (Prep + Cook Time: 2 hours 10 minutes)

In the pot of Ninja Foodi, mix together the water, broth, lemon juice, lemon juice, dill and lemon zest. Arrange the salmon fillets on top, skin side down and sprinkle with salt and black pepper. Close the Ninja Foodi with crisping lid and select "Slow Cooker". Set on "Low" for 1-2 hours. Press "Start/Stop" to begin cooking. Open the lid and serve hot.

Keto Clam Chowder

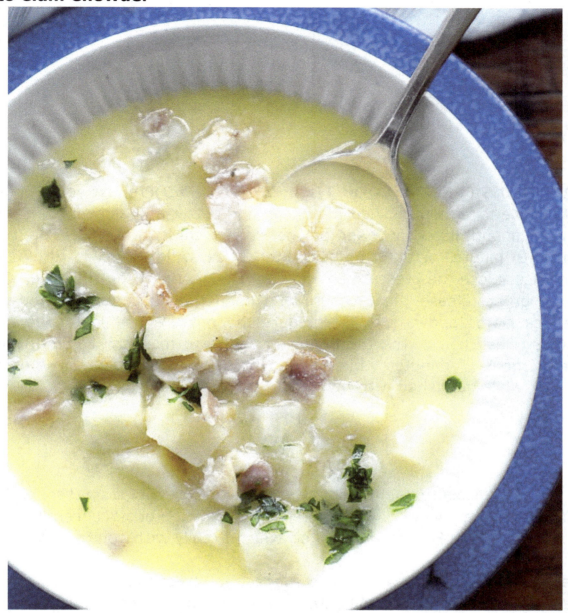

INGREDIENTS (6 Servings)

  4 slices (4.2 oz) of bacon, chopped

4 tablespoons of unsalted butter

1 white onion, diced

2 celery stalks, diced

2 garlic cloves, minced

3 cups of diced turnips

1 teaspoon of sea salt
Few sprigs of fresh thyme
1/4 teaspoon of black pepper
A cup of clam juice 1 lb of clams Optional
1/4 teaspoon of cayenne
2 (10 oz) cans of baby clams, boiled (reserve juice)
1 1/2 glasses of heavy cream

DIRECTIONS (PREP + COOK TIME: 25 MINUTES) Preheat your Foodi on sauté mode for a minute. Add the bacon and butter and allow it to fry for 5 minutes or until its crispy. Add onions, celery, garlic, and spices. Sauté for another 3 minutes or until the spices tenderize. Add the diced turnips and clam juice. Close the pressure lid and cook on low mode for a minute. Once cooked quick release the pressure and open the lid carefully. Add your littleneck clams and cream. Stir. Sauté the mixture on high mode for 4 minutes. Mash half of the turnips using a tomato masher. Let the turnips simmer for 5- 7 minutes while stirring frequently. Serve your Keto clam chowder while garnished with thyme.

Conclusion

Did you take pleasure in attempting these brand-new and tasty dishes?

Sadly we have actually come to the end of this recipe book concerning using the fantastic Ninja Foodi multi-cooker, which I really wish you taken pleasure in.

To enhance your health we want to suggest you to combine exercise as well as a dynamic way of life along with adhering to these amazing dishes, so as to emphasize the improvements. we will be back soon with more and more appealing vegetarian recipes, a large hug, see you soon.

A information can be obtained
w.ICGtesting.com
d in the USA
7062254020621
3LV00014B/43

9 781008 951273